Healthy Lungs Care Guide
Handbook
{Best for Smokers}

By **CYNTHIA LEONARD**

INTRODUCTION:

Understanding the Importance of Lung Health

For general well-being and quality of life, lung health is vital.

Here is a quick summary of its significance:

Breathing: The act of taking in oxygen and releasing carbon dioxide via the lungs is essential to life. Effective gas exchange, which transfers oxygen to the circulation and eliminates waste gases, is ensured by healthy lungs.

Physical Performance: Being physically active requires having optimal lung function. Stamina, endurance and general performance in sports and exercise are all enhanced by good lung health.

Immune Defence: The lungs serve as a defence against allergies, pollutants and airborne viruses. By capturing and eliminating dangerous chemicals, a functioning respiratory system aids in the defence against respiratory infections and illnesses.

Quality of Life: A number of lung conditions, including lung cancer, chronic obstructive pulmonary disease (COPD) and asthma, may have a major negative influence on day-to-day functioning and quality of life. Preventing or minimising these diseases via lung health maintenance may enhance overall health.

Heart Health: By guaranteeing that the bloodstream receives an appropriate amount of oxygen, healthy lungs promote heart function.

Heart problems including heart failure and pulmonary hypertension may be brought on by poor lung health.

Longevity: A healthy lung environment is essential for long life and good ageing. People may lower their chance of acquiring chronic respiratory disorders and their related problems by maintaining healthy lung function.

Environmental Impact: Smoking, air pollution, and workplace dangers are some of the environmental elements that have an impact on lung health. Cleaner settings and the adoption of behaviours that limit exposure to respiratory dangers are key components of lung health promotion.

Early Detection: Regular screenings and evaluations of lung health may help identify respiratory disorders early on and manage them, which can improve prognosis and treatment results.

Encouraging lung health by lifestyle decisions, environmental awareness and medical treatments is important for preserving good health and lowering the incidence of respiratory disorders.

Purpose of this Handbook

This handbook's major goal is to provide everyone, especially smokers, all the knowledge they need to keep their lungs in good condition while continuing in the lifestyle.

It seeks to inform people about the many kinds of cigarettes that are available, the safety precautions that should be taken while smoking and useful advice and guidelines for lung care.

People who are aware of these factors may prioritise lung health and reduce the hazards of smoking by making well-informed choices.

CHAPTER 1:

Types of Cigarettes - From Most Toxic to Less Toxic

Overview of Cigarette Composition

Cigarettes are intricate devices made of different materials that are meant to make it easier to burn and breathe in tobacco smoke. Although the precise makeup may vary across brands and varieties, the basic elements of a cigarette usually consist of:

Tobacco: The main component of cigarettes is tobacco, which is derived from the tobacco plant's leaves. Various tobacco kinds may be utilised, such as burley, oriental and flue-cured varieties, each of which adds unique flavours and qualities to the smoke.

Chemicals: To improve flavour, fragrance and burning qualities as well as control the delivery of nicotine, cigarette producers often add a variety of chemicals. Sugars, flavourings, humectants *(to retain moisture)*, and chemicals *(to regulate combustion and boost smoke production)* are a few examples of these additions.

Paper: The thin paper that covers cigarettes acts as the outer layer. Chemical treatments may be applied to the paper to regulate its rate of combustion and guarantee even burning.

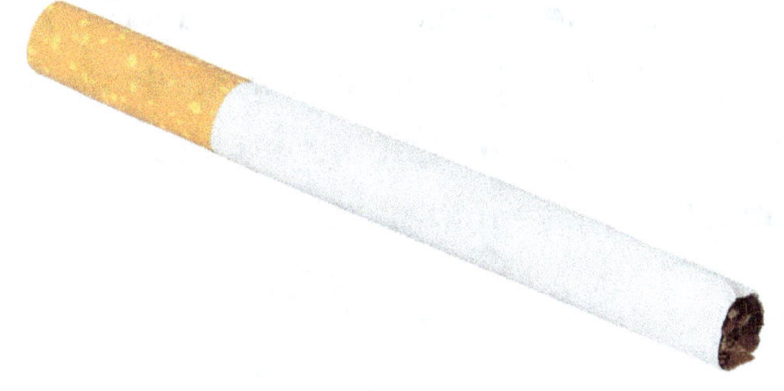

Filter: A cellulose acetate or other material-based filter is found in many cigarettes. The purpose of filters is to limit the amount of tar and other dangerous materials that smokers inhale by trapping some of them in the smoke.

Adhesives: The tobacco mix, paper, and filter parts of the cigarette are held together using a variety of adhesives.

Ash: When the tobacco in cigarettes burns, ash is produced. The remaining inorganic components that are left behind after combustion make up this ash.

Tobacco smoke emits hundreds of compounds while it burns, many of which are toxic to human health. These include the highly addictive drug nicotine, the combination of chemicals known as tar, carbon monoxide, formaldehyde, acrolein, benzene and a host of other substances, some of which are poisonous or carcinogenic.

Do know that the content of cigarettes is regulated in many nations and initiatives like public health campaigns, product standards and tobacco control laws have been implemented in an attempt to lessen the hazardous ingredients in cigarettes.

In spite of these efforts, tobacco smoke and its harmful components continue to be the world's top causes of avoidable mortality from smoking, mostly because of the health concerns involved.

Ranking by Toxicity:

Traditional Cigarettes

Combustible cigarettes, another name for traditional cigarettes - are tobacco products that are smoked by burning the tobacco and breathing in the smoke.

Typically, they are made of a filter and shreds of tobacco leaves wrapped in paper.

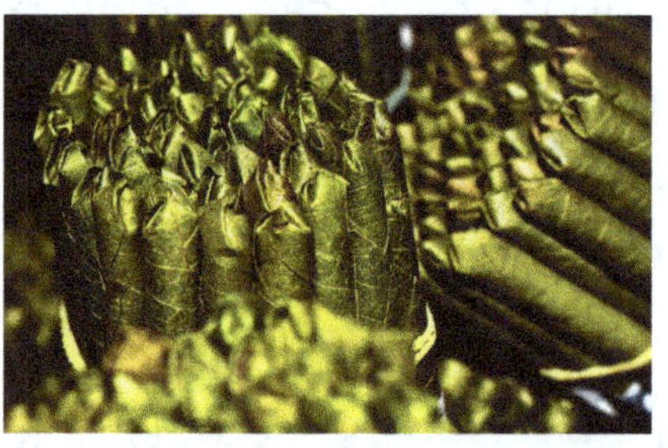

The tobacco burns when it is burned, releasing smoke that contains hundreds of additional compounds, many of which are toxic and cancer-causing, along with nicotine. Although traditional cigarettes have been a common smoke for generations, their well-established harmful health effects—such as an increased risk of heart disease, lung cancer and respiratory problems—have drawn more and more attention to them.

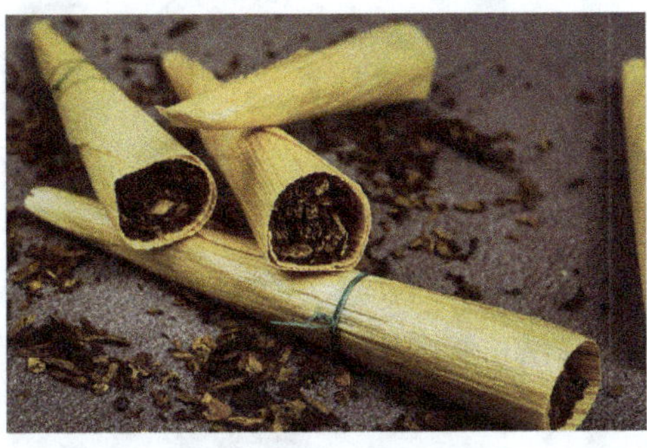

Usage rates have been declining in some regions due to public health campaigns, smoking cessation programmes and the rise of alternative nicotine delivery systems like electronic cigarettes, traditional cigarettes are still widely used worldwide despite growing awareness of these risks.

Menthol Cigarettes

Menthol-containing cigarettes are a particular kind of cigarette that includes menthol, which may be synthetic or obtained from peppermint oil. In addition to providing a cooling effect, menthol softens the harshness of tobacco smoke, making inhalation simpler.

Because of their comparatively softer flavour and experience, these cigarettes have been widely used for many years. But because of

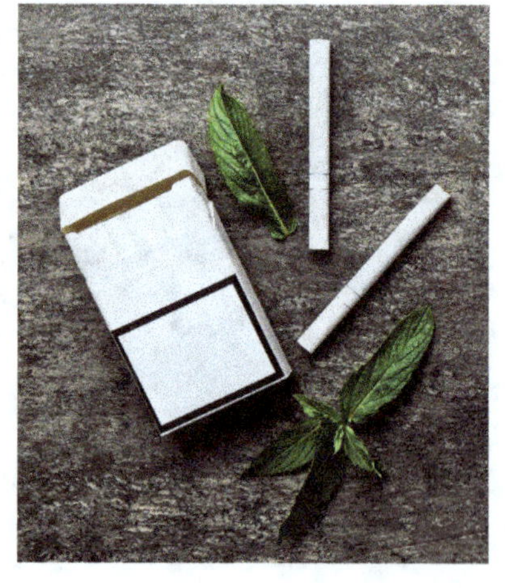

worries about their possible health effects—especially with regard to addiction and their attraction to younger smokers—they have generated debate.

These concerns have led to attempts in certain jurisdictions to restrict or outright prohibit menthol cigarettes.

Light Cigarettes

Light cigarettes, often referred to as low-tar or mild cigarettes, were brought to the market in response to worries about the negative consequences of smoking on one's health. Because there is less tar and nicotine in the smoke, these cigarettes are supposed to provide a softer smoking experience.

Light cigarettes are designed to provide smokers a possibly "safer" option by lowering their exposure to dangerous chemicals while maintaining the enjoyment of smoking.

Cigarette filters are perforated to dilute smoke, manufacturers use tobacco blends with reduced nicotine and tar content and ventilation holes are added to the filter to enable more air to mingle with the smoke to obtain the **"light"** classification. The intended health advantages of light cigarettes, however, may be countered by smokers who inadvertently adjust for their lower nicotine consumption by smoking more often, taking longer puffs or plugging ventilation holes with their fingers, according to study.

Studies have shown that light cigarettes are not as effective as normal cigarettes in lowering the health hazards connected with smoking, despite marketing promises to the contrary. Indeed, several studies indicate that those who smoke light cigarettes can be as susceptible to smoking-related illnesses as those who consume normal cigarettes.

Regulatory bodies across the world have restricted the use of phrases like **"light"** or **"low-tar"** in cigarette marketing due to worries about deceiving customers. To dispel the myth that lite cigarettes are safer than normal cigarettes, several countries have outlawed the use of these terminology completely.

Electronic Cigarettes (e-cigarettes or vapes)

Electronic cigarettes, sometimes called vapes or e-cigarettes are battery-operated devices that vaporise liquids that include flavourings, nicotine and other substances.

They resemble regular cigarettes or pens and they come in a variety of sizes and forms. As an alternative to smoking regular cigarettes, e-cigarettes have grown in popularity. The liquid is heated to generate vapour, which users inhale.

The following are some salient features of electronic cigarettes:

Parts: Usually, an e-cigarette has four parts: a mouthpiece for inhaling the vapour, a cartridge or tank to contain the e-liquid, a heating element *(atomizer or coil)*, and a battery.

E-liquids: Also referred to as vape juice or e-liquid, this liquid solution used in e-cigarettes typically includes flavourings, propylene glycol, glycerin, nicotine and other substances. There are e-liquids with and without nicotine and different amounts of nicotine.

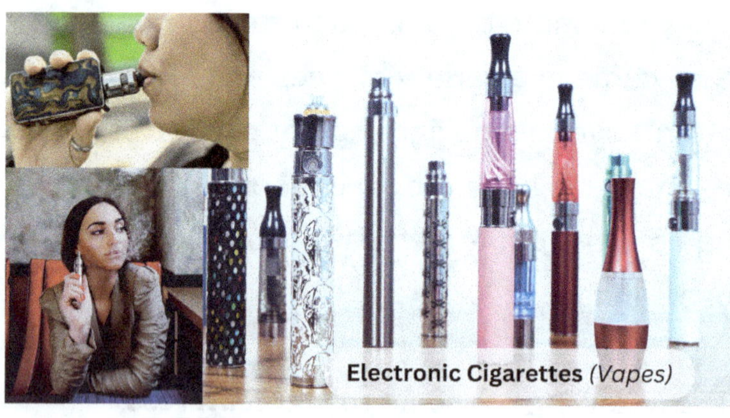

Electronic Cigarettes *(Vapes)*

Vaporisation: The heating element of the device is powered by the battery when the user turns it on, which causes the e-liquid to evaporate. After that, the user inhales the vapour, which fills their lungs with flavourings and nicotine.

Flavours: There are many different flavours available for e-liquids, such as fruit, candy, dessert, menthol and tobacco. Variety in flavours has been a major role in the attractiveness of vaping, especially for younger consumers.

Health Concerns: E-cigarettes do have certain health concerns, despite its frequent marketing promotion as a safer option to conventional smoking. Harmful substances included in vaping aerosol, including nicotine, heavy metals, volatile organic compounds and ultrafine particles, may negatively impact the cardiovascular and pulmonary systems.

Regulation: Each nation and jurisdiction has its own regulations on e-cigarettes. Ad limitations, flavour prohibitions and age restrictions are just a few of the stringent laws that have been put in place in many nations. **The Food and Drug Administration** (FDA) in the **US** is in charge of regulating e-cigarettes and associated goods.

Controversy: Public health professionals, legislators and advocacy organisations have been deeply divided over e-cigarettes. Advocates contend that they have the potential to enhance public health outcomes by assisting smokers in reducing or quitting their tobacco use. However, detractors point out that vaping may have long-term health consequences, especially for young people, and that e-cigarettes might act as a gateway to tobacco usage.

Popularity: E-cigarettes are becoming more and more well-liked, particularly among youth. Teens and young adults' usage of e-cigarettes has drawn criticism since some research points to an increase in nicotine addiction and lung damage from vaping.

Even if e-cigarettes may have certain benefits over conventional smoking, research and discussion on their long-term health consequences and influence on public health are still continuing. It's critical that consumers consider the advantages and disadvantages of vaping and keep up with new research on the subject.

Herbal Cigarettes

Without tobacco, herbal cigarettes are produced from a blend of different herbs or other plant material. Since they don't contain nicotine or other dangerous substances that are usually included in tobacco products, they are often promoted as a healthier option to conventional tobacco cigarettes.

These cigarettes are often marketed as a tool to help people quit smoking or as a means to lessen the negative consequences of tobacco use. *It's crucial to remember that even if herbal cigarettes don't contain nicotine, smoking anything may still be harmful to your respiratory system since it releases smoke and other combustion byproducts into the air.*

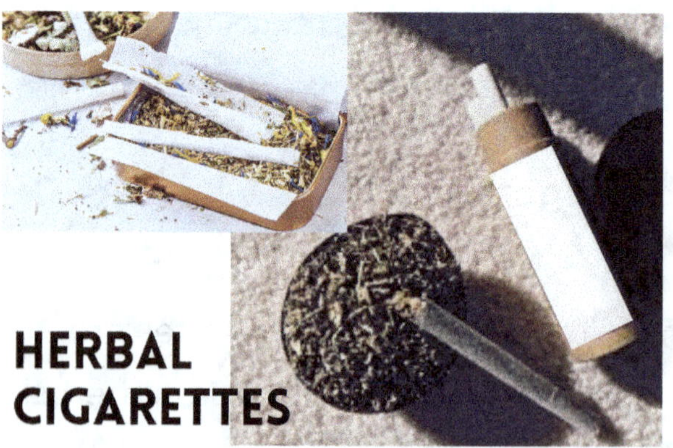

Herbal cigarettes often include a variety of medicinal plants, mint, clover and lemongrass as ingredients. When smoking herbal cigarettes, it's important to exercise caution nevertheless, since some individuals may still react negatively to the smoke or develop respiratory problems.

Safety and effectiveness of herbal cigarettes might differ since they are not subject to the same government health agency regulations as tobacco products.

Before using herbal cigarettes, it is always essential to speak with a healthcare provider, particularly if you are attempting to stop smoking or have any underlying medical concerns.

CHAPTER 2:

Understanding Lung Health

Anatomy and Function of the Lungs

The process of respiration, which involves exchanging carbon dioxide and oxygen between the body and the environment, is carried out by the lungs -one of the essential organs. The rib cage surrounds them, keeping them safe within the thoracic cavity.

Now let's examine their structures and roles:

Lung Anatomical Structure

Lobes: There are lobes in each lung. The left lung contains two lobes *(upper and lower)*, but the right lung has three *(upper, middle and lower)*. There are lesser divisions inside these lobes.

Airways that branch out and into the bronchial tree carry air into and out of the lungs. The trachea is the starting point and it splits into the left and right major bronchi as well as lesser bronchi and bronchioles.

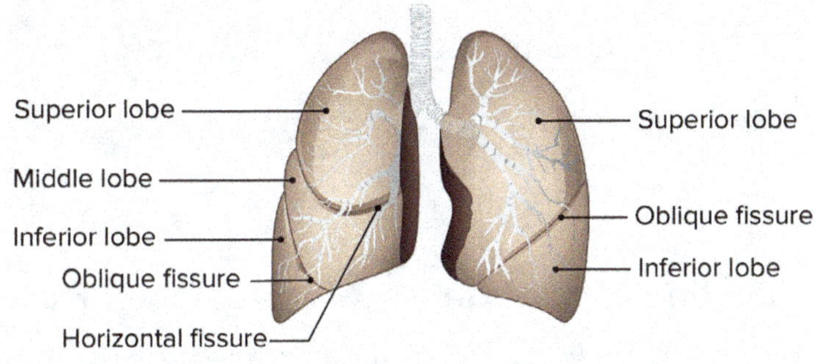

Alveoli: The small air sacs where gas exchange takes place are located at the end of the bronchial tree. Because blood capillaries round these sacs, carbon dioxide may escape and oxygen can enter the circulation.

Pleura: The pleura is a double-layered membrane that covers the lungs. The outside layer, known as parietal pleura, borders the chest cavity, while the inner layer, known as visceral pleura, clings to the lungs.

A little quantity of fluid, found in the pleural cavity, which sits between these layers, lessens friction during breathing.

Function of the Lungs - *Gas Exchange:* The lungs' main job is to make it easier for the blood to exchange carbon dioxide and oxygen with the outside environment. After entering the alveoli and diffusing into the capillaries, oxygen from breathed air attaches itself to haemoglobin in red blood cells.

Simultaneously, circulatory carbon dioxide diffuses into the alveoli for exhalation.

The flow of air into and out of the lungs is referred to as ventilation. The diaphragm and intercostal muscles flex during inhalation *(spiration)*, widening the thoracic chamber and lowering air pressure, which allows air to enter the lungs quickly. These muscles relax during expiration and the lungs' elastic rebound aids in the release of air.

pH regulation: By regulating blood carbon dioxide levels, the lungs contribute to the body's pH homeostasis. A combination of carbon dioxide and water may produce carbonic acid, which changes the pH of blood.

The lungs regulate breathing depth and pace to improve the body's acid-base equilibrium.

Defence Mechanism: The respiratory system has defence systems to keep the lungs safe from irritants, germs and foreign particles. These include immune cells that aid in the battle against infections, cilia that remove debris from the airways and mucous membranes that trap particles.

The lungs are intricate organs that are necessary for breathing, exchanging gases, preserving the pH balance in the body and shielding it from dangerous chemicals. They are vital to the continuation of life because of their complex structure and effective operation.

Common Lung Conditions

Among the most common lung diseases are the following:

Chronic asthma is characterised by inflammation and constriction of the airways, which may cause coughing, shortness of breath, chest tightness and wheezing.

Emphysema and Chronic Bronchitis are two disorders that are included in the progressive lung illness known as chronic obstructive pulmonary disease or COPD. It obstructs airflow and makes breathing difficult.

Pneumonia is an infection of the lungs that may be brought on by viruses, bacteria or fungus. It results in inflammation of one or both lung's air sacs, which may cause symptoms including fever, chills, coughing and dyspnea.

Inflammation of the Bronchial Tubes, which transport air to the lungs, is known as bronchitis. While chronic bronchitis is a kind of

COPD characterised by a productive cough lasting at least three months for two consecutive years, acute bronchitis is often caused by viruses and resulting in a persistent cough.

Pulmonary Embolism (PE): A blood clot that enters the lungs from another area of the body—usually the legs—causes Pulmonary Embolism or PE. Abrupt dyspnea, chest discomfort, fast heartbeat and haemorrhaging are some of the symptoms.

The term **Interstitial Lung Disease (ILD)** describes a collection of lung conditions marked by inflammation and scarring of the tissue that surrounds the lungs' air sacs, known as the interstitium.

Because of this scarring, oxygen cannot easily enter the circulation, which results in symptoms including coughing, dyspnea and a reduced ability to tolerate physical activity.

Lung Cancer: Uncontrollably growing abnormal cells in one or both lungs may result in lung cancer. Although it is often linked to smoking, it may also happen to non-smokers. Coughing, chest discomfort, dyspnea, blood in the cough and inadvertent weight loss are some of the symptoms.

Pulmonary Fibrosis: This condition causes the lung tissue to thicken and scar, which reduces lung function and makes breathing harder. Although the aetiology is sometimes unclear *(idiopathic)*, exposure to pollutants in the environment, certain drugs or connective tissue problems may all be contributing factors.

Cystic Fibrosis (CF): The hereditary illness known as Cystic fibrosis (CF) affects the lungs and other organs, resulting in the creation of thick, sticky mucus that clogs airways and causes difficulty breathing. It raises the possibility of respiratory issues and lung infections.

Sleep Apnea: During sleep, people with sleep apnea have shallow or periodic breathing pauses. It may result in increased risk of cardiovascular issues, poor focus and exhaustion throughout the day.

There are several more illnesses that might have an impact on respiratory health; these are only a few instances of prevalent lung ailments.

Effects of Smoking on Lung Health

Smoking affects the structure and function of the lungs, having a significant and negative impact on lung health.

Some of the main outcomes are:

Diminished Lung Function: Smoking impairs the lungs' alveoli or air sacs and airways, which results in a reduction in lung function. Conditions such as chronic obstructive pulmonary disease (COPD), in which breathing becomes difficult due to limited airflow, may arise from this.

Enhanced Risk of Respiratory Infections: Smokers have a higher risk of developing respiratory illnesses including pneumonia and bronchitis. Smoking damages airways, which creates a perfect habitat for germs and viruses to proliferate and lowers the immune system's capacity to fight off illnesses.

Chronic Bronchitis: Smoking irritates the bronchial passages, which results in excessive mucus production and persistent inflammation, which causes chronic bronchitis. This illness, sometimes referred to as chronic bronchitis, results in a chronic cough and trouble cleaning the airways.

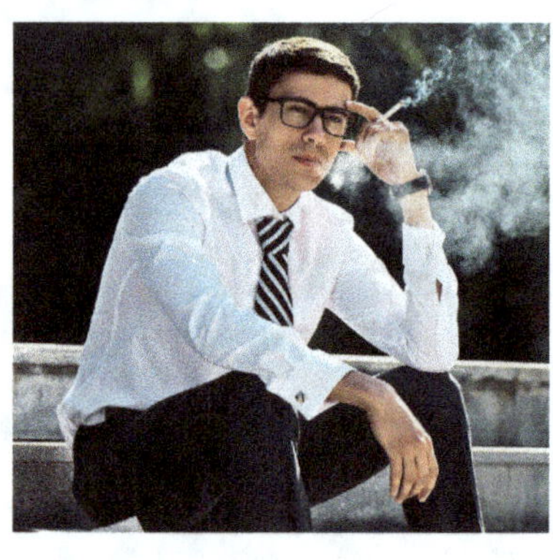

Emphysema: Smoking damages the lungs' alveoli, which are in charge of exchanging carbon dioxide and oxygen. Emphysema, a lung illness that progresses over time and is characterised by shortness of breath and decreased exercise tolerance, is the result of this damage.

Elevated Risk of Lung Cancer: Smoking is the main global cause of lung cancer, responsible for most occurrences. Tobacco smoke contains carcinogens that harm lung cells' DNA, causing unchecked cell division and tumour development.

Asthma Severance: Smoking aggravates asthma symptoms and raises asthma attack frequency and intensity. In nonsmokers as well, secondhand smoke exposure may exacerbate asthma symptoms, especially in young children.

Reduced Wound Healing: Smoking hinders the body's capacity to heal wounds, especially lung injury. This may impede the healing process after lung surgery and other respiratory ailments.

Smoking Accelerates Lung Ageing: Smoking causes early lung damage and a reduction in lung function by hastening the lungs' normal ageing process. This may cause symptoms including dyspnea and decreased endurance during physical activity, even in very young people.

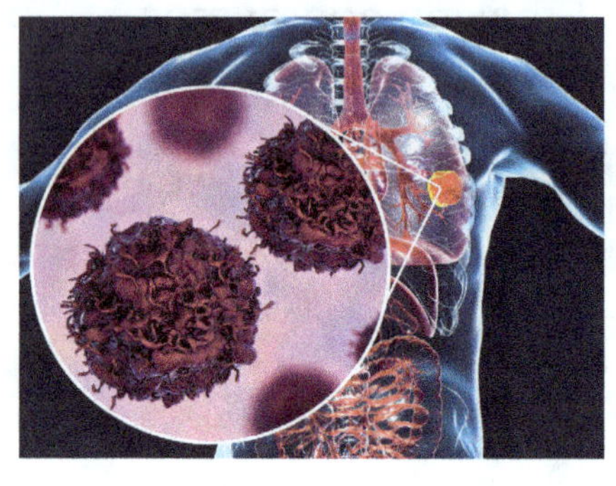

Smoking has a significant detrimental impact on lung health and general well-being, making it one of the world's biggest avoidable causes of disease and death. The single best thing people can do to protect their lungs and lower their chance of smoking-related illnesses is to give up smoking.

Tips for Active Smokers to Protect and Cleanse the Lungs

Here are some suggestions for current smokers who want to lessen the harm and improve lung health:

Give Up Smoking: This is the most crucial action. Consult medical experts, programmes to help you stop smoking or support groups for assistance.

Keep Yourself Hydrated: Water thins mucus and facilitates the removal of toxins from the lungs.

Maintain a Healthy Diet: Eat plenty of fruits and vegetables, such as kale, spinach, oranges and berries, that are high in antioxidants.

Antioxidants may assist in preventing the harm that smoking causes.

Exercise on a Regular Basis: Exercise helps enhance lung capacity and function. On most days of the week, try to get in at least 30 minutes of moderate activity.

Engage in Deep Breathing Exercises: These breathing techniques may enhance lung function and capacity. Try breathing exercises like pursed-lip breathing or diaphragmatic breathing.

Minimise Your Exposure to Secondhand smoking: Since secondhand smoking may harm your lungs as well, try to avoid it.

Minimise Your Exposure to Air Pollution: Try to keep your home and automobile exhaust, industrial emissions and interior pollutants like mould and dust as low as possible.

Think About Air Purifiers: To assist reduce pollutants and enhance the quality of the air within your house, install air purifiers.

Get Regular Check-ups: Schedule routine examinations and lung function testing with your healthcare practitioner.

Explore Herbal Remedies: Eucalyptus, peppermint and ginger are a few herbs that may improve lung health and calm the respiratory system. Before utilising any herbal treatments, however, speak with a healthcare provider, particularly if you use medication or have any pre-existing illnesses.

Reduce Your Exposure to Respiratory Irritants: Reduce your exposure to allergies, fumes and harsh chemicals.

Maintain Good Hygiene: Wash your hands often to lower the chance of respiratory infections, which may make lung issues worse.

Use a Humidifier: Humidifiers provide moisture to the air, which helps relieve breathing and soothe sore airways.

Seek Medical Advice: You should see a physician right away if you have chronic respiratory problems or if you have concerns about the health of your lungs.

CHAPTER 3:

Lifestyle Changes

Diet and Nutrition

For general health, it is important to keep the lungs healthy so food and nutrition are important for lung health.

These food recommendations and nutrients may support the health of your lungs:

Foods High in Antioxidants: Antioxidants help shield lung tissue from harm brought on by 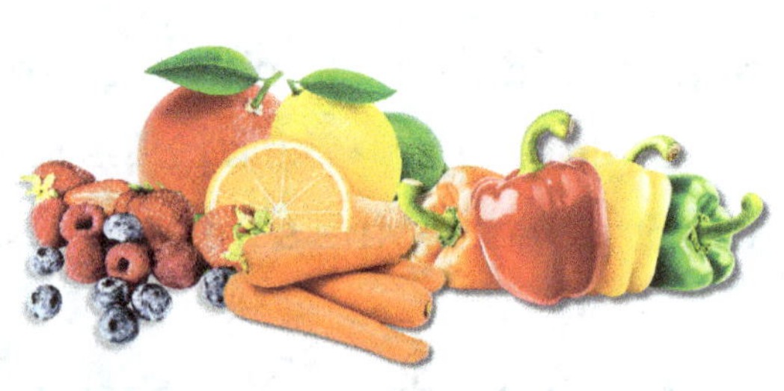 pollution and free radicals. Consume a diet rich in fruits and vegetables, such as carrots, bell peppers, leafy greens, citrus fruits and berries.

Omega-3 Fatty Acids: Rich in flaxseeds, chia seeds, walnuts and fatty fish like trout, salmon and mackerel, omega-3 fatty acids contain anti-inflammatory qualities that may be good for lung health.

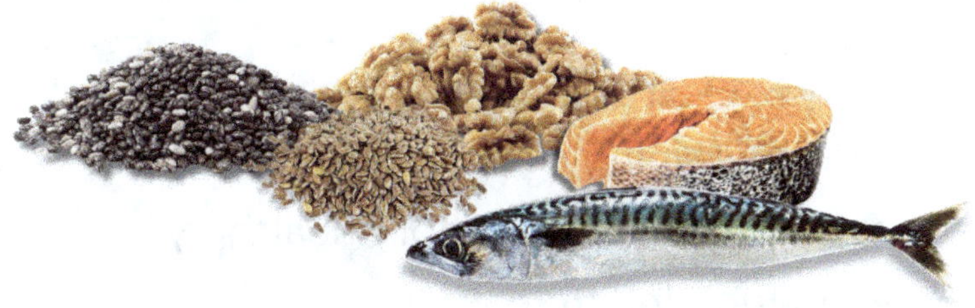

Vitamin C: Rich in immune system support and potential protection against respiratory infections, vitamin C may be found in citrus fruits, strawberries, kiwi, bell peppers and broccoli.

Vitamin E: Packed with antioxidants that shield lung cells from harm, vitamin E is found in nuts, seeds, avocados and spinach.

Beta-Carotene: The body transforms beta-carotene, which is found in foods like carrots, sweet potatoes, spinach and kale, into vitamin A. To keep lung tissue healthy, vitamin A is necessary.

Onions and Garlic both include sulphur-containing chemicals that have been shown to improve respiratory health by lowering lung inflammation.

Herbs & Spices: Anti-inflammatory and antioxidant qualities of oregano, ginger and turmeric are well-known and may be advantageous to lung health.

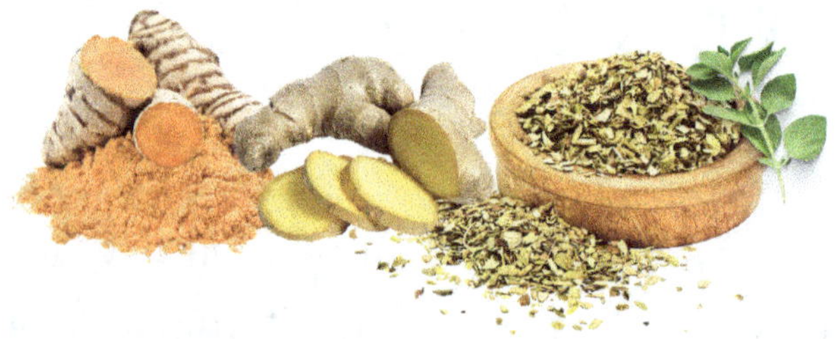

Green Tea: Green tea has anti-inflammatory properties and antioxidants called catechins that may help protect lung tissue.

Water: Maintaining enough hydration lowers the risk of respiratory infections by keeping lung mucus thin and easy to remove.

Avoid Hazardous Substances: Restrict or stay away from foods and drinks that may be harmful to your lungs, such as processed foods rich in trans fats, sugary drinks and too much alcohol.

Also, abstain from smoking, secondhand smoke and pollution from the environment.

To maintain total wellbeing, do note that although a nutritious diet may promote lung function, it's

Exercise and Physical Activity

Physical activity and exercise are essential for keeping the lungs healthy and the respiratory system functioning as a whole.

Some ways that physical activity supports lung health:

Increased Lung Capacity: By strengthening the respiratory muscles and boosting the effectiveness of oxygen exchange in the lungs, regular exercise helps to increase lung capacity.

This implies that each breath you take will allow your lungs to absorb more oxygen and release more carbon dioxide.

Increased Respiratory Efficiency: Physical activity encourages the lungs to function at a higher level. Your breathing rate rises during physical exercise, which facilitates better oxygen intake and delivery to the muscles. This may eventually result in improved respiratory health in general.

Decreased Risk of Respiratory Illness: Engaging in regular exercise can lower the chance of contracting respiratory infections like the flu or the common cold as well as respiratory diseases like asthma and chronic obstructive pulmonary disease (COPD).

Exercise helps the body fight off infections by enhancing lung function and fortifying the immune system.

Enhanced Lung Function in Chronic illnesses:
Exercise may still be helpful for those who
have long-term respiratory illnesses like COPD
or asthma.

A healthcare provider should be consulted
before beginning any fitness programme,
although many individuals with these
problems may safely exercise, which can help
improve lung function, lessen symptoms and
improve overall quality of life.

Weight Control: Maintaining a healthy weight
is mandatory for lung health and may be
achieved by regular exercise. Breathing
becomes more difficult and puts pressure on
the lungs when one is overweight.

By engaging in physical activity and exercise to
maintain a healthy weight, you may lessen the
strain on your lungs and minimise your chance

of developing respiratory issues linked to obesity.

Better Cardiovascular Health: Exercise is good for the heart and blood vessels, which helps to maintain lung health. Walking, jogging, swimming and cycling are examples of aerobic exercises that increase cardiovascular fitness and facilitate the heart's ability to pump blood more effectively, supplying oxygen-rich blood to the body's tissues, including the lungs.

Increased General Fitness: Frequent exercise increases stamina and general fitness, which eases daily tasks and lessens weariness. A physically fit body puts less burden on the respiratory system since your lungs have to work harder to perform daily chores.

Aim for at least 150 minutes of moderate-intensity aerobic activity or 75 minutes of vigorous-intensity activity each week, together with muscle-strengthening activities on two or more days, in order to benefit from exercise for lung health.

Always pay attention to your body, begin slowly if you've never exercised before and see a doctor if you have any questions or concerns about underlying medical issues.

Stress Management

Maintaining healthy lungs involves various factors, including stress management. Chronic stress can negatively impact overall health, including respiratory health.

To manage stress, practise deep breathing exercises, regular exercise, mindfulness and meditation and yoga. Maintain a healthy lifestyle by eating a balanced diet, getting enough sleep and avoiding substances like tobacco and excessive alcohol.

Seek social support by surrounding yourself with supportive friends and family members. Time management is essential to reduce feelings of being overwhelmed and allocate time for relaxation and leisure activities.

Limit exposure to stressful situations by setting boundaries, learning to say NO, or making lifestyle changes. If stress becomes overwhelming or unmanageable, seek professional help from a mental health professional. Therapy or counselling can provide strategies to cope with stress more effectively.

By incorporating these practices, you can improve your lung function, reduce stress and maintain a healthy lung environment.

CHAPTER 4:

Smoking Reduction Strategies:

Gradual Reduction

A smoking reduction technique called **"Gradual Reduction"** entails progressively cutting down on cigarettes smoked until quitting is accomplished. Although this strategy would seem more sensible and manageable than giving up suddenly, medical specialists disagree on how beneficial it is.

The following factors and advice should be taken into account while using gradual decrease as a smoking cessation method in order to protect your lungs:

Have a Well-defined Reduction Strategy:

Define a precise timetable and reduction plan. For instance, try cutting down on cigarettes smoked by a certain quantity every day or every week until you smoke none at all.

Track Your Development: Maintain a notebook to record your smoking behaviours and progress. This might support your motivation and accountability.

Determine Triggers: Keep an eye out for circumstances, feelings or actions that set off the desire to smoke. To address these triggers without turning to cigarettes, try finding other coping strategies or diversion.

Use Nicotine Replacement Therapy (NRT): To assist manage withdrawal symptoms while you progressively cut down on smoking, think about utilising nicotine patches, gum, lozenges or other NRT products. These may be especially useful in making the switch to reduced nicotine levels easier.

Seek Support: Share your reduction objectives with loved ones, a medical professional or pals. Having encouragement and support may help to streamline the process.

Use Stress Reduction Strategies: Smoking is often used as a stress-reduction strategy. Examine other approaches to reducing stress, such as exercising, meditating, doing deep breathing exercises or taking up a hobby.

Modify Your schedule: Make a change to your schedule to help break the link between smoking and particular activities. *For example,* consider drinking tea or taking a stroll in place of smoking if you usually have coffee in the morning.

Celebrate Your Success: Whether it's going a week without smoking or cutting down on smoking a day, acknowledge and treat yourself when you meet your goals.

Remain Upbeat and Persistent: Recognise that stopping smoking is a difficult process with potential obstacles. Remain committed to your objective and don't let brief failures deter you.

Think About Professional Assistance: You may want to see a healthcare provider if you're having trouble cutting down or quitting smoking on your own. In addition to offering customised guidance and support, they might also suggest other tools or drugs to help with quitting smoking.

Nicotine Replacement Therapy (NRT)

People who smoke may benefit from **Nicotine Replacement Therapy (NRT)**, which gives them nicotine in a form that is safer than cigarettes. It entails employing nicotine delivery devices, such as patches, gum, lozenges, inhalers or nasal sprays to give regulated dosages of nicotine free of the dangerous compounds present in tobacco smoke.

By lessening the cravings and withdrawal symptoms linked to giving up smoking, NRT increases the likelihood of a successful cessation.

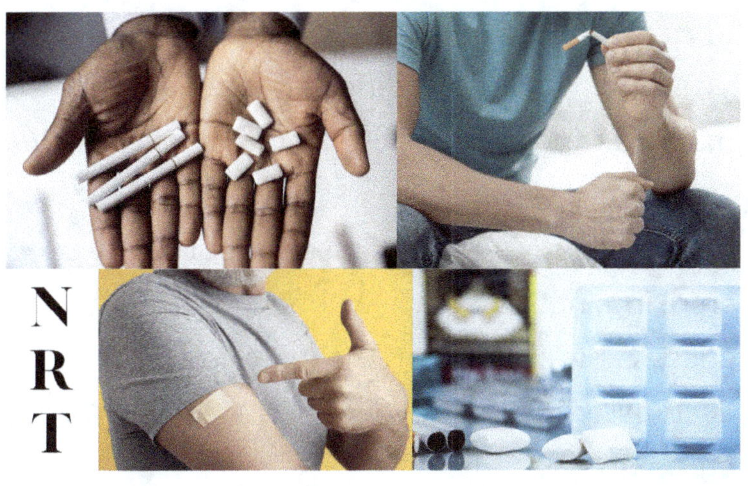

The idea behind NRT is to taper down the dose gradually over time in order to lessen nicotine dependency. This makes it simpler for people to stop smoking by assisting them in managing withdrawal symptoms including irritation, anxiety, problems focusing and cravings.

In many nations, NRT products may be purchased over-the-counter, while others might need a prescription. They may be taken alone or in conjunction with other cessation strategies like counselling or support groups.

They are available in different strengths to meet varying degrees of nicotine dependency.

Although NRT may be a useful tool for quitting smoking, not everyone will benefit from it and success often relies on the individual's circumstances and level of dedication to stopping.

Furthermore, NRT medicines continue to provide nicotine, so if they are not taken as prescribed, dependence may develop.

CHAPTER 5:

Lung Cleansing Techniques

Deep Breathing Exercises

Here are Steps to a Basic Deep Breathing exercise:

Choose a Comfortable Position: Take a seat or lay down where you feel most at ease. *You have two options:* lay down on your back with a cushion under your head and legs or sit upright on the ground or a chair.

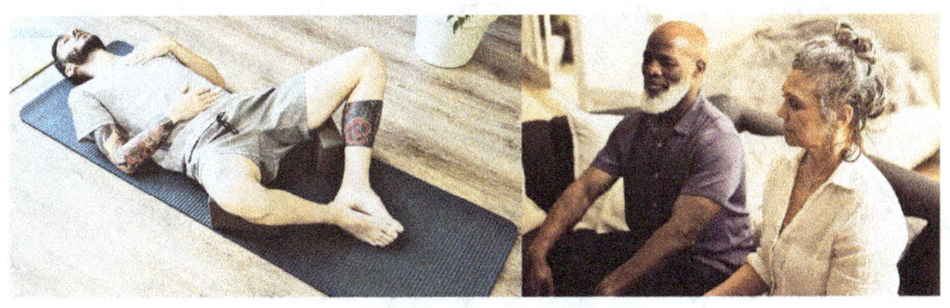

Deep Breathing Exercise

Shut your eyes and spend a few minutes letting your body relax. Starting with your head and working your way down to your toes, release any tension that may be stored in your muscles.

Breathe Deeply and Slowly Through Your Nose: Start by inhaling deeply and slowly through your nose. Pay attention to fully filling your lungs with air. As you breathe in, feel your abdomen and chest become larger.

Hold Your Breath: After taking a big breath, hold it for a little while. As you become more used to the activity, progressively increase the time from the initial, comfortable range of 3 to 5 seconds.

Breathe Out gently and thoroughly Through Your Mouth: Release your breath gently and thoroughly through your mouth after holding it.

- Concentrate on getting all the air out of your lungs. As you release the breath, feel your belly and chest tighten.

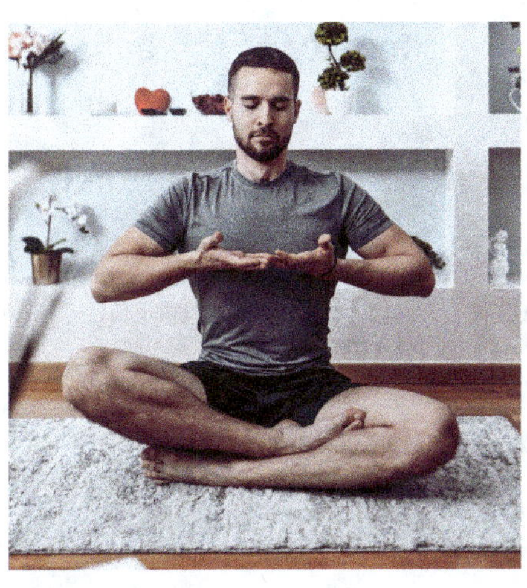

Repeat: Make numerous rounds of this deep breathing cycle, trying to stay in the zone for at least 5 to 10 minutes. Pay attention to the rhythm of your breathing and make an effort to regulate and smooth each inhale and expiration.

Remain Aware: Throughout the workout, pay attention to your breathing and your body's feelings. With every breath, pay attention to how your lungs expand and contract and note any changes in your level of relaxation.

Increase Intensity progressively: As you become more comfortable with deep breathing, you may add breath-holding exercises or longer inhalations and exhalations to progressively up the intensity of the activity.

Remain Consistent: Practise deep breathing on a regular basis to get the advantages of lung cleaning. Whether you do them in the morning, at regular intervals throughout the day or just before bed, make it a point to include deep breathing exercises in your daily regimen.

Steam Inhalation

A common technique for clearing the lungs and reducing respiratory symptoms is steam inhalation.

This is how it works and should be done safely:

Boil Water: To begin, bring a pot or kettle of water to a boil. For extra advantages, you may also add herbs or essential oils, like eucalyptus, peppermint or chamomile to the water.

After the water has boiled, gently transfer it to a basin that can withstand heat. Take care not to burn yourself.

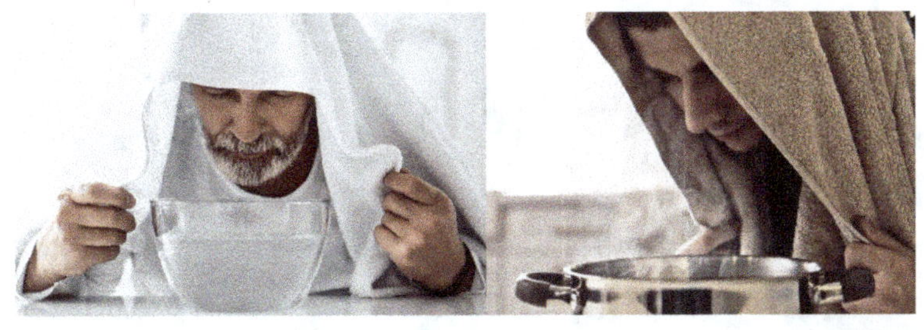

***Optional-* Add Essential Oils:** To the hot water, add a few drops of essential oil if you're using them. Tea tree, Peppermint and Eucalyptus essential oils may assist relieve congestion and strengthen the respiratory system further.

Make a Tent: To prevent burns, place your face over the bowl but at a safe distance. To capture the steam, cover your head and the bowl with a cloth to form a tent.

Inhale Steam: Spend a few minutes taking deep, full breaths of the steam via your nose. *Additionally*, you have the option to choose between breathing via your mouth and nose.

Take Rests: Take rests as required if the temperature is too high or unpleasant.

use Caution: To prevent burns, use caution while approaching the hot water.

Benefits of Inhaling Steam:

Clear Congestion: Steam facilitates the evaporation of mucus and phlegm from your respiratory tract.

Reduce Sinus Pressure: Steaming may help open the nasal passages and reduce sinus pressure.

Wet Dry Airways: It may aid in wetting dry airways, relieving discomfort and dry coughing.

Reduce Respiratory Symptoms: Inhaling steam may temporarily reduce symptoms of respiratory disorders such as tightness in the chest, wheezing and coughing.

Not everyone may find steam inhalation to be appropriate. Before attempting steam inhalation, those with certain respiratory disorders, such as asthma, should exercise caution and speak with a healthcare provider.

Take caution to avoid being burned by the steam or hot water. If you feel any pain or unfavourable responses, cease right away and if needed, get medical help.

Hydration and Detoxification

Lung cleansing is important for maintaining respiratory health, especially for those exposed to pollutants or those with respiratory conditions.

Strategies include staying hydrated by drinking at least 8 glasses of water daily, practising deep breathing exercises like diaphragmatic breathing, pursed lip breathing and alternate nostril breathing, also engaging in regular physical activity such as walking, jogging, cycling and swimming.

Smoking and secondhand smoke can damage the lungs and increase the risk of respiratory diseases like **COPD** and lung cancer. Quitting smoking is the most effective way to improve lung health, while minimising exposure to air pollutants is essential.

Avoiding areas with heavy traffic, industrial sites and poor ventilation can help reduce exposure.

A balanced diet rich in fruits, vegetables, whole grains and lean proteins provides essential nutrients and antioxidants that support lung health.

Antioxidants like vitamin C, vitamin E and beta-carotene protect lung tissue from oxidative damage caused by pollutants and toxins.

Herbal remedies like ginger, turmeric, licorice root and eucalyptus may support lung health and detoxification, but it's important to consult with a healthcare professional before using them.

Maintaining good posture allows for full lung expansion during breathing, which aids in clearing out toxins and promoting optimal lung function.

These strategies should not replace medical treatment for respiratory conditions, but they can support lung health and detoxification.

Herbal Remedies and Supplements

The effectiveness and safety of herbal medicines and supplements might differ greatly, despite the fact that they are often used in traditional medical practices for a variety of reasons, including lung health.

Before beginning any new herbal cure or supplement regimen, always get medical opinion, particularly if you are using medication or have pre-existing health issues.

Having stated that, the following herbs and substances are often linked to promoting lung health:

Peppermint:

Peppermint is well-known for its capacity to relieve congestion and widen airways.

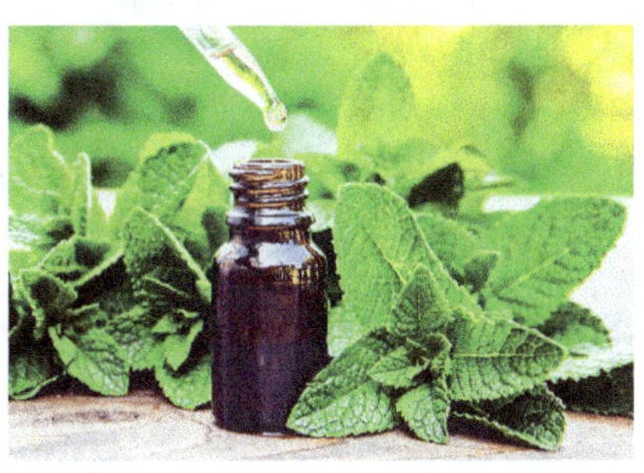

Because of its natural decongestant properties, menthol may help relieve the symptoms of respiratory diseases including bronchitis and asthma.

Eucalyptus: To reduce congestion and enhance breathing, eucalyptus is often used in inhalation treatments.

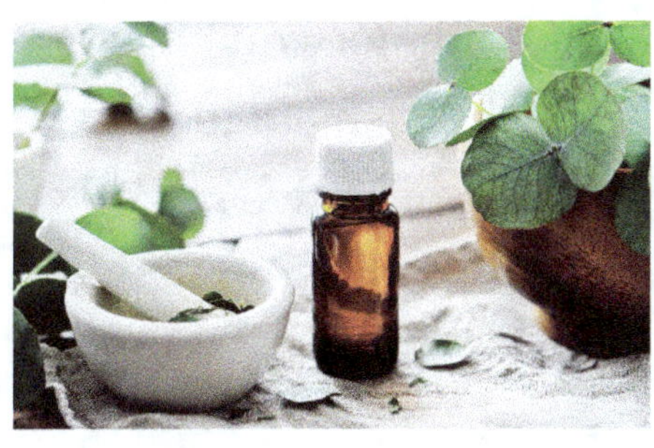

Cineole-containing chemicals found in its oil have expectorant qualities that help break up mucus and make coughing easier.

Ginger: Ginger may help maintain lung health because of its anti-inflammatory and antioxidant qualities. It may enhance respiratory health by lowering airway inflammation.

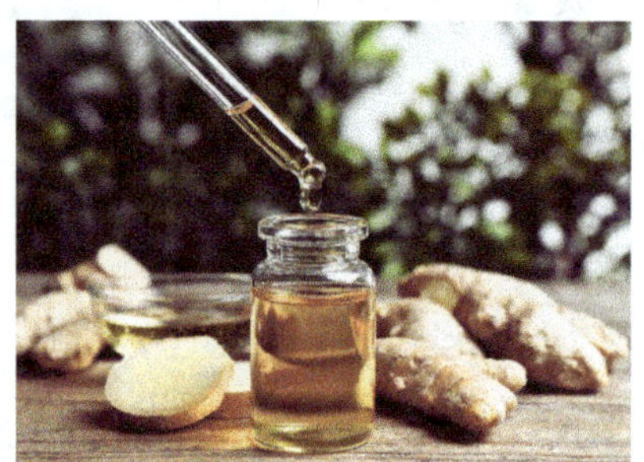

Turmeric: The key ingredient in turmeric, curcumin, has antioxidant and

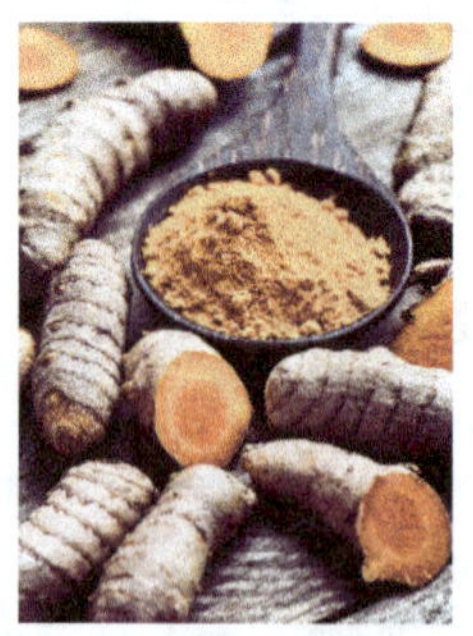

anti-inflammatory qualities that may help shield lung tissue from oxidative stress and inflammation-related damage.

Garlic: Allicin, one of the chemicals found in garlic, has antibacterial and anti-inflammatory qualities. By lowering inflammation and thwarting respiratory infections, it could promote lung health.

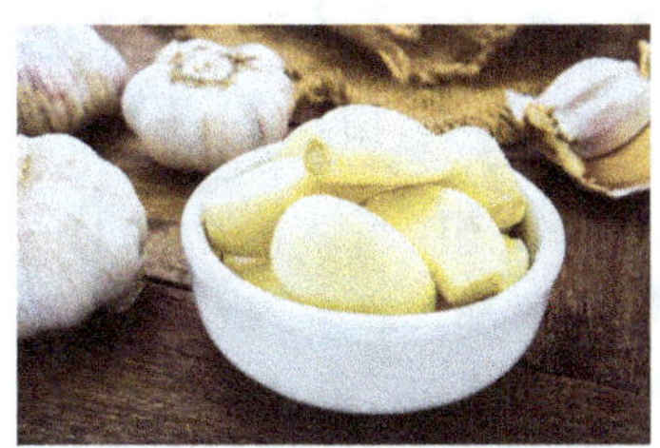

Licorice Root: Traditionally, coughing fits and respiratory tract irritations have been soothed by using licorice root. It could encourage sputum production and lessen irritation.

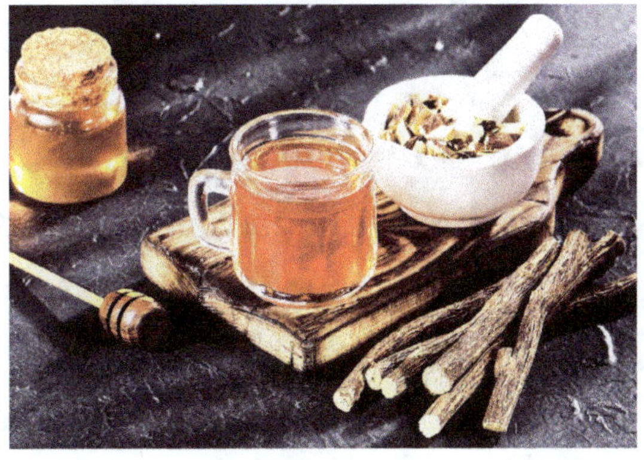

Licorice Root

Vitamin C: As an antioxidant and immune system booster, vitamin C helps maintain lung function by defending against oxidative stress. Citrus fruits, strawberries, bell peppers and broccoli are foods high in vitamin C.

Vitamin D: A lack of vitamin D has been connected to a higher risk of lung conditions and respiratory infections. Maintaining sufficient amounts of vitamin D via supplementation and exposure to sunshine may aid in maintaining lung health.

Omega-3 fatty acids: Due to their anti-inflammatory qualities, omega-3 fatty acids may help lessen lung inflammation and enhance respiratory health. Walnuts, flaxseeds, and fatty fish are good sources of omega-3 fatty acids.

N-acetylcysteine (NAC): NAC is a supplement with mucolytic capabilities, which means it thins and breaks down mucus to facilitate its removal from the respiratory system. For respiratory diseases such as cystic fibrosis and chronic obstructive pulmonary disease **(COPD)**, it is sometimes used as a supplemental treatment.

You should take supplements and herbal treatments with caution and under a doctor's supervision, particularly if you are on medication or have pre-existing medical issues. Always adhere to the suggested doses and use guidelines.

CHAPTER 6:

Building a Support System

Seeking Professional Help

For general respiratory health, getting expert assistance is essential for keeping healthy lungs.

Here's 'how-to' for locating the appropriate experts and resources:

First and foremost, make an appointment with your **Primary Care Physician (PCP)**. They may evaluate your general health, which includes lung function and provide advice on lifestyle modifications and preventative actions to maintain the health of your lungs.

A Pulmonologist is a medical professional that your PCP may recommend if you have particular concerns about your lung health or respiratory problems including asthma, COPD *(chronic obstructive pulmonary disease)* or lung infections. These experts specialise in the identification and management of lung conditions.

Healthcare workers with training in **Respiratory Therapy** are experts in diagnosing and treating breathing issues. To enhance lung function, they may instruct patients on methods like inhaler usage, breathing exercises and pulmonary rehabilitation.

Allergist / Immunologist: An allergist or immunologist may assist in the diagnosis and treatment of allergies or immunological disorders that impact your respiratory system. To reduce symptoms and enhance lung health, they could suggest immunotherapy, allergy testing or medication.

Programmes for Quitting Smoking: One of the most essential things you can do to safeguard the health of your lungs is to stop smoking. To assist you in effectively quitting, a lot of healthcare professionals provide smoking cessation programmes or may direct you to other services like support groups, counselling, or nicotine replacement treatment.

Nutritionist / Dietitian: Eating a balanced diet is important for keeping the lungs in good condition. A nutritionist or dietitian may design a customised diet plan that includes foods high in antioxidants, vitamins and minerals, which are proven to improve respiratory function, to promote lung health.

Exercise physiologist / Physical therapist: Exercise on a regular basis may enhance respiratory health in general and lung function in particular. Whether you want to improve lung capacity, boost endurance or manage a respiratory illness, an exercise physiologist or physical therapist can create a safe and efficient training programme just for you.

Mental Health Professional: Stress, depression and anxiety may worsen respiratory symptoms and have an adverse effect on lung health. Seeking assistance from a psychologist, psychiatrist or counsellor may help if you're having mental health issues.

They can provide coping mechanisms and emotional support to enhance your general wellbeing.

Support Groups and Local Resources: Making connections with others who have gone through similar things may be a great way to get support and motivation. Seek out

regional support groups or online respiratory
health forums where you may exchange
experiences, learn from others and get advice.

*You may take proactive measures to preserve healthy
lungs and maximise your respiratory well-being by
getting expert assistance and making use of the
resources that are available.*

Support Groups and Resources

In order to preserve respiratory health, prevent
lung illnesses and provide assistance to those
coping with lung-related problems, support
groups and resources for healthy lungs may be
very important.

A list of some of these resources and support groups:

Lung Association of America (ALA): A
multitude of resources are available from the

American Lung Association to help you keep your lungs healthy, such as information on lung health education, programmes to help you quit smoking, air quality efforts and assistance for those with lung disorders.
https://www.lung.org

COPD Foundation:

The COPD Foundation offers advocacy, education and support to people with chronic obstructive pulmonary disease **(COPD)** and those who care for them. They provide tools including patient support programmes, internet forums and instructional materials.
www.copdfoundation.org is the website.

The ATS (American Thoracic Society):

The mission of the American Thoracic Society is to advance critical care, sleep and pulmonary medicine. They provide resources, such as

patient education materials, support groups, and details about lung disorders and treatments to both patients and healthcare professionals.
https://www.thoracic.org

Alliance Against Lung Cancer:

The Lung Cancer Alliance offers advocacy and assistance to those who are impacted by lung cancer. They include educational materials, support groups, and details on available treatments as well as other resources for patients, carers and medical professionals. www.lungcanceralliance.org is the website.

The Foundation for Pulmonary Fibrosis:
People with pulmonary fibrosis, a degenerative lung illness, may find information and assistance from the Pulmonary Fibrosis

Foundation. They provide instructional resources, information on clinical trials, research updates and support groups. www.pulmonaryfibrosis.org is the website.

Alpha-1 Basis:

The primary goal of the Alpha-1 Foundation is to provide assistance to those who suffer with alpha-1 antitrypsin insufficiency, a hereditary disorder that may result in liver and lung damage. They provide educational materials, support groups and research updates, among other services to patients, carers and healthcare professionals. https://www.alpha1.org

Online Communities of Support: Online communities are provided by platforms like PatientsLikeMe and Inspire, which enable people to connect with others going through comparable lung health issues, exchange stories and get support.

Websites: www.patientslikeme.com and www.inspire.com

Local Medical Facilities and Hospitals:

For those with lung disorders, a lot of hospitals and health facilities provide support groups and educational initiatives. To find out what options exist in your region, get in touch with your local healthcare professionals.

People may get helpful knowledge, direction and encouragement to maintain healthy lungs or successfully manage lung-related diseases by using these support groups and services.

It's important to maintain knowledge, ask for help when you need it, and give lung health first priority in your diet and medical attention.

Engaging Family and Friends

Engaging family and friends in promoting healthy lungs can create a supportive environment for everyone involved. To do this, lead by example by practising healthy lung habits yourself, such as quitting smoking, exercising regularly and avoiding exposure to pollutants.

Educate your family and friends about the importance of lung health and the benefits of healthy behaviours like exercise and proper nutrition. Openly communicate about lung health within your social circle, creating a safe space for everyone to discuss their concerns and experiences.

Organise group activities that promote lung health, such as group workouts, hikes or bike rides to bond and support each other.

Create a smoke-free environment, encouraging smokers to quit or refrain from smoking in shared spaces. Promote clean air by using air purifiers, avoiding indoor pollutants and advocating for policies that reduce air pollution.

Stay informed about the latest research and recommendations related to lung health, sharing relevant information with your family and friends to empower them to make informed decisions.

Celebrate milestones and successes in your journey toward better lung health, acknowledging and celebrating these achievements together.

When needed, seek professional help, such as consulting with a doctor, pulmonary specialist, or smoking cessation counsellor.

By engaging family and friends in promoting healthy lungs, you can create a supportive network that fosters positive habits and encourages everyone to prioritise their respiratory health.

CONCLUSION

Commitment to Lung Health, Future Goals and Maintenance

To ensure optimal lung health, individuals should quit smoking, avoid harmful substances, engage in regular exercise, maintain a healthy diet, stay hydrated, practise good posture and breathing techniques, schedule regular health check-ups with healthcare providers, stay updated on vaccinations, manage chronic conditions like asthma or COPD and incorporate mindfulness breathing and stress management techniques into their daily routine.

Giving up smoking is the most crucial step to improve lung health and reduce the risk of lung disease, cancer and other respiratory issues.

Exposure to harmful substances, such as secondhand smoke and air pollution, should be minimised. Regular exercise can strengthen lungs and improve their efficiency.

A balanced diet rich in fruits, vegetables, whole grains, lean proteins and healthy fats is essential for overall health.

Staying hydrated is essential for maintaining lung function including regular health check-ups with healthcare providers to detect potential issues early and discuss respiratory symptoms. Managing chronic conditions through medication, lifestyle modifications and regular monitoring can also help manage symptoms effectively.

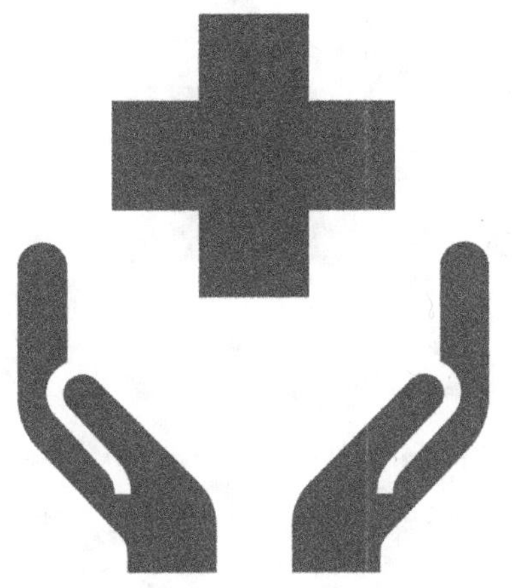